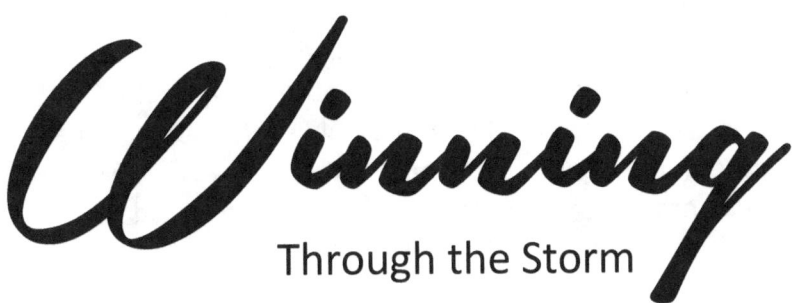

Winning
Through the Storm

The Healing Process
TONYA FREEMAN

Winning Through the Storm 2

Table of Content

Winning Through the Storm 4

Acknowledgements

Everyone needs a great support system and these individuals have stood beside me through it all.

Kelly Thompson, what can I say!!! Thank you for reading to me, thanks for praying with me, and thanks for holding my hand during my most difficult time. I love and appreciate your heart towards me. Thanks for always dropping what you are doing to be there for me.

My siblings, my sister, Tamika Freeman-Belk and my brother Paul Freeman, III never left my side, and for that I am forever grateful.

Ronald Frye and Brian Price are simply amazing. These two men support me unconditionally and I appreciate them both. Thanks for co-parenting our children with me. You guys rock!!

Last, but certainly not least, my wonderful children, Antonio, Destinee and Madison, I live because of all of you. Thank you for being patient with me. I don't always get it right as your mom, but I try my best to live a good life before you guys. I love you forever. I am super proud of each and every one of you. My desire for you is for you to be the best "YOU" that you can be, whatever your best may be.

To all of my readers who are currently experiencing sickness and disease in their body, know that you don't have to take it. God took it, so you don't have to, I understand your pain. I command your body to line up with the Word of God and that you are made whole in the name of Jesus.

Dedication

I dedicate this book to two special people in my life, first, my mother Sandra Ann Hunt, who passed on January 8, 1996 of Cancer. Her strength was amazing. She showed me how to endure, she showed me how to be strong, and she showed me how to be a good mother. Second, is my grandfather, Walter Hunt, Sr., he was the first guy that I ever loved. This man raised me, he spoiled me as best as he knew how, he provided for me and he protected me. I was his "Shug", I miss him so much. He passed on June 15, 2006. I am forever grateful for my mother & my grandfather. Because of them, I am!

Winning Through the Storm 8

CHAPTER ONE
My Story

Have you ever been so sick that you wanted to die? My first headache started when I was just 18 years old; the year was 1996; I was fresh out of high school. I didn't think much of the headaches until they kept coming back.

At this point in my life, I had already given birth to my son, who was then one year old and very active. Being sick was definitely an interruption in my household. I was also a freshman at the University of the District of Columbia and working full-time, I didn't have time to be sick. At first, I ignored the headaches & continued with life as usual, but, the headaches kept coming back. I finally went to my primary doctor and they simply prescribed me pain medicine. The pain medicine didn't relieve the headaches, so I would have to lie in bed until they went away. Some days, I would miss work or school because the headaches were so bad.

This was a lot for an 18 year old to deal with. The headaches would ease up and life was back on track; so I thought.

One year later, we found out my mother had cervical cancer. I was 19; this was too much to deal with. I was shocked and upset. Life as I knew it would never be the same. Will she die? So many questions and no answers. All of these thoughts and stress triggered headaches to resurface.

My insurance, at the time was Kaiser, so it was never a problem getting an appointment. Again, I went to see my physician but this time, I asked if I could see a specialist. *You must take responsibility and control of your own health.* During this time, I was in nursing school at the University of the District of Columbia, and had been doing some research on migraines and the different types of headaches. My doctor agreed, it was time for me to see a neurologist and two weeks later I did just that.

Well, it was just as frustrating seeing the specialist as it was seeing my primary care physician. I still didn't get any answers. The Neurologist just gave me more medicine. I stayed on the medication for about five years before they switched me to another, because it was not keeping the migraines under control. I was on beta blockers, calcium blockers and depression medication, all used to treat migraines and not the other symptoms.

Fast forward to 2003. The migraines started to take a turn for the worse. My neurologist put me on seizure meds to prevent the attacks and remove all of the other meds because of the severity of the headaches. Let me explain how it feels when my body is being attacked: I can't hear any noise; I must lay completely still; I can't talk; I can't smell anything; I'm nauseous; I have a loss of appetite; I lose weight; I am unable to care for my kids.

As of the writing of this book, they have gotten worse. I have seen specialists after specialists to no avail; no cure or relief. I have relied strictly on my faith to get me through this difficult time.

When in crisis, the migraine typically last 6-8 weeks. During this time I experience a migraine every day lasting 10 hours a day during those weeks, with no relief in sight; nothing to subdue the pain.

Other issues came as a result. I can't eat, sleep, lie down in my bed; I can't care for my children which is the worst feeling as a mom. My children are cared for outside the house by their father because I just couldn't do it.

My last crisis happened at the beginning of November 2012, just before Thanksgiving. I thought to myself, "God, what do I do?" He said, "What you've always done!!!"

And so I did! I knew that I had only a few weeks before things got bad, so I started spending every second with my kids. I started preparing for the storm. Once Thanksgiving came, I was house bound because the pain had taken over. Depression tried to set in but I was armed with my confession, "I have the mind of Christ". A week later, things began to get worse and I had to be hospitalized. This time I had swelling on my brain which required steroids by IV. Boy was I upset! Anybody that knows me knows, I don't like being hospitalized.

Once I was discharged, I had to go home for a 7-day course of an intense regimen of steroids to relieve the swelling and pressure on my brain. This was 3 or 4 weeks prior to Christmas. My youngest daughter Madison kept telling me all she wanted for Christmas was for me to feel better. This crushed me because she was only seven years old and instead of thinking about toys, school, running and playing, she was worrying about her mother health.

I guess by now you are wondering how I qualify to write a book on the process of healing if I haven't been healed. Good question, and I'm glad you asked. The answer, however, is simple. I believe the Word of God! *"Surely he took up our pain and bore our suffering, yet we considered him punished by God, stricken by him, and afflicted. But he was pierced for our transgressions, he was crushed for our iniquities; the punishment that brought us peace was on him, and by his wounds we are healed."* *Isaiah 3:4-6* Therefore, while I am waiting on the manifestation of my healing, I confess the Word of God regardless of how I feel. I meditate on His Word and His love and I trust the process.

Winning Through the Storm 16

CHAPTER TWO

What to Do When You Are Going Through

The greatest challenge, when you are going through an attack on your health is to have the mindset to confess what you know the Word of God says about your situation. That's why I recommend that you have, on hand, CD's and DVDs on healing; have a song in your spirit that you can sing when the pain is bad. Listen to the cd's and sing the songs over and over again.

In addition, it's also imperative that you have a good support system. The enemy came to me so many nights telling me that I had nobody; he even tried to tell me to commit suicide. I told him I will live and declare the work of The Lord! When nobody is there with you, you must know that God will never leave you nor forsake you. *Deuteronomy 31:6* **Believe** me, I understand; its hard, I've been there, but God loves you and so do I. You will get through this. Remember, God is not a respecter of person; He did it for me and He will do it for you. Don't give up on yourself; He never gave up on you.

He endured the cross with you in mind, Glory to God for that! You are special to Him. You must know that death isn't an option and you will not die before your time. That has to be your confession. *You are needed and your assignment and purpose isn't fulfilled.* This is what He kept telling me, so I'm telling you.

People are counting on us. Don't grow weary; just magnify Him during this process. I promise it will get better. All storms come to an end! Praise God!

Preparation for the storm

If you know you experience the same illness prepare for the attack. For me, my family knows that my crisis will last 6-8 weeks. I have a little time before my body completely shuts down; therefore, I get prepared for the worst of the storm. I contact my family and friends to let them know the attack has started. My job is made aware of what is going on, so I begin to organize my workload just in case I will be out of work for a lengthy timeframe. I contact my children's schools to inform them of what is occurring. I notify my friends asking them, if they plan on visiting me, not to wear any scents or bring any food with a smell because this will either trigger another attack or make the attack worse. So preparation is huge in the healing process. During a weather related storm we run out to get batteries, milk, eggs, bread, etc. Likewise, when it comes to Heath related storms, we need to have, our Word, CDs, family and friends, prepared food, account number accessible for bill payments, pharmacy numbers, physician numbers, etc.

Remember the enemy comes to steal our confession, by His stripes we are healed, healing belongs to the children of God. Stand on His Word

The Storm

Sometimes I have warning signs to let me know that I am about to experience an attack. The first and main sign is a migraine. Most people can have a migraine and it doesn't bother them, but for me, when I get one, it is the beginning of a 2-3 month battle. I have been diagnosed with Cluster Headaches, which are different from migraines and very rare. I have an extreme case. It tells me to roll up my sleeve, put the gloves on because we are in for a fight. After the first attack, I experience a migraine at least four times throughout the day, nonstop without relief for 6 weeks. During the storm, I miss at least one month of work, so I am very grateful for an understanding company. My children aren't home with me because I am unable to care for them, so they are sent with their father's during this time. I am basically home alone dealing with this and totally relying on God to get me through this storm.

The Aftermath

After every storm there is an aftermath. There is a cleanup process. For my household I must repair things. Play catch up on bills because I was out of work. Go grocery shopping, clean entire house, wash clothes; begin to restore my body back to where it was. For me, my body still experiences symptoms of my crisis, not migraines, but other symptoms such as body weakness, loss of appetite so even though the crisis is over the aftermath is still in effect.

Continue to make declarations over your life. Remove all negativity from your life; don't allow anyone or anything to interrupt the healing process.

Accomplishments

- Certified Zumba Instructor
- Personal Trainer
- Began teaching Zumba classes
- Established Free&Fit, LLC
- Free&Fit Boot camp
- Promotion & Increase on Job
- Pursuing Degree
- Attended children school events/activities
- Published First Book

CHAPTER THREE
Healing Confessions and Scriptures

ealing is the children's bread, therefore I cancel every sickness, disease, infirmity, and plot that the enemy has to cause me or my family to be in the bondage of sickness. The bible says: "Where the spirit of the Lord is, there is liberty." The spirit of the Lord lives in me and is upon me; therefore I have been liberated. I am saved. I am Sozo, which means saved, healed, and delivered. I am delivered from all the attacks of the wicked one and I walk in continual health.

In the days of the children of Israel, God brought them out of Egypt with not one sick or feeble one among them. Since then, He has given us a new covenant with even better promises than that. One of those promises is that everything that Jesus took on His back, I no longer have to take.

Jesus, I glorify Your name and worship who You are. I thank You for what You did on that cross for me over 2,000 years ago. You bore my sicknesses and by Your stripes, I was healed.

Therefore, body, in the name of Jesus, I command you to

line up with God's word: I am healed! I speak to every muscle, tissue, ligament, bone, my blood, and every part of my body from my head to my toes, and I call you whole right now in Jesus name. I call you healed and whole.

Father, I thank You for the healing anointing that flows through my body that protects me from all sickness, hurt and disease in Jesus name.

Prov. 4:23; 10:27

I fear the Lord and I prolong my days. I keep my heart with all diligence for out of it flows the issues of life.

Prov. 13:12; Prov. 14:27, 30

My desire is only of the Lord and it is a tree of life. I fear the Lord and He is my fountain of life. I have a sound heart and it is the life of my flesh.

Prov. 17:22; Prov. 18:20-21

I have a merry heart and it does good like a medicine. My belly is satisfied by the fruit of my mouth, and with the increase of my lips I am filled. Death and life are in the power of my tongue. I speak the life-giving words of God and I receive life and health in my body.

Isa. 53:4-5; 1 Peter 2:24

Jesus Christ has borne my sicknesses and carried my pain. He was stricken, smitten of God and afflicted for me. He was wounded for my transgressions and He was bruised for my guilt and iniquities. The chastisement needed to obtain peace and well-being for me was upon Him, and with the stripes that wounded Him, I am healed and made whole. I now have perfect health in my body.

Matt. 6:10; Gal. 2:20; 1 John 4:17

The will of God is done on earth as it is done in heaven. There is no sickness in heaven; therefore, I am not sick at all on the earth. Jesus was never sick on this earth. Jesus is in me and His life flows in me. As He was in the world so am I in this world. I am healthy as Jesus was healthy upon this earth.

Matt. 8:17; 1 John 3:8; Acts 10:38

Jesus destroyed the works of the devil, which were diseases, sicknesses, and bodily infirmities; therefore, all the works of the devil upon my body are destroyed and I have perfect health in Jesus Christ.

Matt. 12:37; Heb. 12:2; Mark 11:23; Matt. 10:1; Mark 16:18

I am justified by my words. I have the faith of Jesus Christ in me, for Jesus is in me, and He is the Author and Finisher of my faith. I speak unto the mountains of sickness and disease and they obey my words and leave. I have authority and power over all disease and sickness; I command them to leave and they obey my words. I lay my hands on the sick and they recover.

Mark 9:23; 2 Cor. 1:20

I believe in God and all His promises, and all things are possible unto me. All the promises of God are yes unto me for Christ has paid the price for all of them.

Mark 11:23-24

I believe that all those things I say shall come to pass. All things which I desire, when I pray, I believe that I have received them and I have them.

John 14:13-14

Whatsoever I ask in the Name of Jesus, Jesus himself does it that the Father may be glorified in the Son. When I ask for anything in the Name of Jesus, Jesus says He will do it.

John 16:23-27; 17:23

The Father loves Jesus Christ and gives Him all that He asks. The Father loves me as much as He loves Jesus and gives me everything that I ask.

Matt. 28:18; Acts 3:16

All authority in heaven and earth is given unto Jesus Christ. I have faith in the power and authority of the Name of Jesus Christ and through His Name I am made perfectly whole.

Rom. 8:11

The Spirit of God who raised up Jesus Christ from the dead dwells in me, and He who raised up Jesus Christ from the dead, also quickens and gives life to my mortal body through His Spirit who now dwells in me.

Rom 10:9,10; Mark 5:23; Acts 14:9

I confess with my mouth the Lord Jesus Christ and believe in my heart that God has raised Him from the dead and I am healed. For with my heart I believe unto righteousness and with my mouth confession is made unto healing and health.

Isa. 58:8; John 17:22; Jer. 33:6

My health springs forth and the glory of the Lord is revealed in me. The Lord brings me health and cure, and reveals unto me the abundance of peace and truth.

Gal. 6:8-9

I sow to the Spirit and reap of the Spirit life everlasting. I sow words of health and healing every day and daily reap health in my physical body.

Heb. 2:14; Col. 2:14-15; Mark 16:17-18

Jesus has destroyed Satan and spoiled all his principalities and powers, and they no longer have any power in me. In the Name of Jesus, I have power over them and over all their works of sickness and disease.

Rom. 10:8

The word is near me, even in my heart and in my mouth; that is the word of faith which I speak.

3 John 2

It is the will of God that I should prosper and be in perfect health even as my soul prospers.

1 Cor 6:19-20; Eph. 3:19

My body is the temple of the Holy Spirit and all the fullness of God dwells in me. I glorify God in my body and in my spirit which are His.

I received healing when I received my salvation. Since I'm no longer under the curse of the law, I am free from the curse of sickness and disease. The Lord is faithful to heal all of my diseases. He removes my sickness and restores me to complete health and wellness.

I release my faith now as I speaking that by Jesus stripes I am healed and confess my total healing from the top of my head to the soles of my feet. My words will come to pass, and I believe that I have my healing now. I stand in faith knowing that no weapons formed against me will prosper.

Scripture References: Galatians 3:13-14, 29; I Peter 2:24; Exodus 15:26, 23:25; Jeremiah 30:17; Isaiah 53:5; Mark 11:23-24; Isaiah 54:17

The Truth of God's Word supersedes facts. I believe the report of God's Word. Isaiah 53:1-6 I shall not die, but live, and declare the works of the LORD. Psalms 118:17 I obtain a good report through the faith that comes through Jesus Christ. Hebrews 11:1-2, Acts 3:16

If you are not saying the same things that Jesus said, don't expect to do the same works that Jesus did.

Your answer in prayer is as close to you, as your confession of God's Word.

Jesus is seated in Heaven "far above all principality and power and might and dominion, and every name that is named" Ephesians 1:21

Jesus has "a name which is above every name", even the name of cancer. Philippians 2:9-11

Jesus Christ said anyone who believes in him will do the same works that he did and even greater works, because he was going to the Father. John 14:12

"Bless the LORD, O my soul, and forget not all His benefits: who forgives all your iniquities. Who heals all your diseases". Psalms 103:2-3

God is my Yahweh Rapha' [Jah-Way Raw-Faw].

The scriptures states that, "as he is, so are we in this world." What actions or works was Jesus doing throughout the Gospels? 1 John 4:17

He was "teaching in their synagogues, preaching the gospel of the kingdom, and healing all kinds of sickness and all kinds of disease among the people". Matthew 4:23

James 5:16, Romans 3:22
My prayers are effectual and avail much, because I am the righteousness of God through faith in Jesus Christ.

Isaiah 55:11
So is My Word that goes out of My mouth: it will not return to Me empty, but it will accomplish what I desire and achieve the purpose for which I sent it.

Proverbs 18:21
The tongue has the power of life and death

Hebrews 4:12

The Word of God is living and powerful

Isaiah 53:5

But he was wounded for our transgressions; he was bruised for our iniquities: the chastisement for our peace was upon him; and with his stripes we are healed.

Galatians 6:9

And let us not be weary in well doing: for in due season we shall reap, if we faint not.

Galatians 3:13

Christ has redeemed us from the curse of the law, being made a curse for use: for it is written, cursed is every one that hangers on a tree:

3 John 1:2

Beloved, I wish above all things that thou may east prosper and he in health even as thy soul prospereth.
And this is the confidence that we have in him, that, if we ask any thing according to his will, he heareth us:

And if we know that he hear us, whatsoever we ask, we know that we have the petitions that we desired of him.
1 John 5:14, 15

For it is God which worketh in you both to will and to do of his good pleasure. Philippians 2:13

He that spared not his own Son, but delivered him up for us all, how shall he not with him also freely give us all things? Romans 8:32

James 1:17
Every good gift and every perfect gift is from above, and comets down from the Father of lights, with whom is no variableness, neither shadow of turning.

Romans 8:31
If God be for us, who can be against us?

Malachi 3:6
For I am The Lord, I change not...,

Isaiah 41:10

Fear thou not; for I am with thee: be not dismayed; for I am thy God: I will strengthen thee; yea, I will help thee; yea, I will uphold thee with the right hand of my righteousness

Deuteronomy 7:15

And The Lord will take away from thee all sickness, and will put none of the evil diseases of Egypt, which thou know east, upon thee.

Jeremiah 33:6

Behold, I will bring it health and cure, and I will cure them, and will reveal unto them abundance of peace and truth.

Psalms 23:1

The Lord is my shepherd; I shall not want.

Psalms 103:3

Who forgiveth all thine iniquities; who healeth all thy diseases.

Psalms 147:3

He healeth the broken in heart, and bindeth up their wounds.

Numbers 23:19

God is not a man that he should lie; neither the son of man that he should repent: hath he said, and shall he not do it? Or hath he spoken, and shall he not make it good?

Jeremiah 29:11

For I know the thoughts that I think toward you, saith the LORD, thoughts of peace, and not of evil, to give you an expected end.

CHAPTER FOUR

The Facts about Migraines

What is a Migraine Headache?

A migraine is an intense throbbing or a pulsing sensation in one area of the head and is commonly accompanied by nausea, vomiting, and extreme sensitivity to light and sound. The attacks can cause significant pain for hours to days.

What is a Cluster Headache?

A cluster headache is a headache that occurs in a cyclical patterns or clusters, which give the condition its name. Cluster headaches are one of the most painful types of headaches. The symptoms can be, restlessness, excessive tearing, redness in your eye on the affected side, drooping eyelid or swelling around your eye on the affected side.

During the attack headaches usually occur every day, sometimes several times a day. A single attack may last from 15 minutes to three hours or longer. An attack period generally lasts from 6 to 12 weeks. Cluster periods may be seasonal, such as every spring or every fall. It normally leaves you exhausted due to the length of time you were in pain.

Cluster headaches typically wake you in the middle of the night with intense pain in or around one eye on one side of your head. These attacks may last from weeks to months. During remission, no headaches occur for months and sometimes years.

Migraines are an extraordinarily common disease that affects 36 million men, women and children in the United States. Almost everyone either knows someone who has suffered from migraine, or has struggled with migraine themselves. According to the Migraine Research Foundation:

- Nearly 1 in 4 U.S. households includes someone with migraine.
- Amazingly, over 10% of the population - including children - suffers from migraine. That's more than diabetes and asthma combined!

- About 18% of American women and 6% of men suffer from migraine.
- Migraine is most common during the peak productive years, between the ages of 25 and 55.
- Migraine tends to run in families. If one parent suffers from migraine, there is a 40% chance a child will suffer. If both parents suffer, the chance rises to 90%.

Many people do not realize how serious and debilitating migraines can be. In addition to attack-related disability, migraine interferes with a sufferer's ability to function in everyday life, whether that is going to school or work, caring for family or enjoying social activities.

- Migraine ranks in the top 20 of the world's most disabling medical illnesses.
- Every 10 seconds, someone in the United States goes to the emergency room with a headache or migraine.
- While most sufferers experience attacks once or twice a month, 14 million people or about 4%

have chronic daily headache, when attacks occur at least 15 days per month.

- More than 90% of sufferers are unable to work or function normally during their migraine.

Migraines are not just a bad headache.

- Migraine is an extremely debilitating collection of neurological symptoms.

- Migraine is a severe recurring intense throbbing pain on one side of the head, although in about 1/3 of attacks, both sides are affected.

- Attacks are often accompanied by one or more of the following: visual disturbances, nausea, vomiting, dizziness, extreme sensitivity to sound, light, touch and smell, and tingling or numbness in the extremities or face.

- In 15-20% of attacks, other neurological symptoms occur before the actual head pain.

- Attacks usually last between 4 and 72 hours.

For many sufferers, migraines are a chronic disease that significantly diminishes their quality of life.

- About 14 million people experience chronic daily headache – when attacks occur at least 15 days per month.
- For more than 90% of all sufferers, migraine interferes with their education, career and social activities.
- Depression, anxiety, and sleep disturbances are common for those with chronic migraine.

Migraine headaches are a public health issue with serious social and economic repercussions.

- American employers lose more than $13 billion each year as a result of 113 million lost work days due to migraine.
- Chronic illness – a category into which migraine can fall - is one of the country's biggest healthcare challenges, and costs an estimated $50 billion per year.
- Migraine sufferers, like those who suffer from other chronic illnesses, face the consequences of high costs of medical services, too little support, and limited access to quality care.

- People with migraine use about twice the medical resources –including prescription medications and office and emergency room visits– as non-sufferers.

Migraines remain a poorly understood disease that is frequently undiagnosed and undertreated.

- Nearly half of all migraine sufferers are never diagnosed.
- The majority of migraine sufferers do not seek medical care for their pain.
- Only 4% of migraine sufferers who seek medical care consult headache and pain specialists.

Yet, in spite of the prevalence of migraines and its serious effect on individuals, families and society, research into the causes and treatment of migraines are severely under-funded.

- At present, NIH funding for migraine research is $15 million - less than 0.03% of the annual NIH research budget.

Children also suffer from migraines.

- The illness often goes undiagnosed in children.

- About 10% of school-age children suffer from migraines.
- Half of all migraine sufferers have their first attack before the age of 12. Migraine has even been reported in children as young as 18 months old.
- Children who suffer are absent from school twice as often as children without migraine.
- Before puberty, boys suffer from migraine more often than girls; as adolescence approaches, the incidence increases more rapidly in girls than in boys.

Migraines disproportionately affect women, with approximately 27 million female sufferers in the United States.

- Three times as many women as men suffer from migraine in adulthood.
- About half of affected women have more than one attack each month, and a quarter experience 4 or more severe attacks per month.
- In childhood, boys are affected more than girls, but after adolescence, when estrogen influence

begins in young girls, the risk of migraine and its severity rises in females.

- More severe and more frequent attacks often result from fluctuations in estrogen levels.

* *Facts gathered from Migraine Research Foundation*
* *National Institute of Health*

Prayer

I thank you God, what you died for I was delivered from. I will live and not die and declare the work of The Lord. God you are my healer, You have set before me life and death, so I choose life. I thank you that I have the mind of Christ and with long life God You will satisfy me and show me how good it is to be saved Lord thank you for restoring my health and for healing me. Thank you God for your peace that surpassing all understanding. Thank you that you are my provider. I received total deliverance in the Name of Jesus. I receive all that I have prayed in Jesus Name. Amen.

About the Author

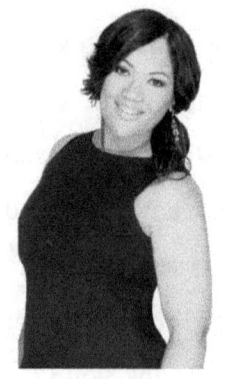

Tonya Freeman is a mother of three, an entrepreneur, and a healthcare manager. She is the founder of FREE & FIT, LLC and is a health and wellness instructor.

Tonya is very passionate towards seeing people advance in every area of their life and she believes that if she can win in life, so can they. Tonya has used her faith for every situation that she has encountered. Her unwavering faith has allowed every situation to turn around in her favor.